M K HIGGINS

Fibromyalgia: Journey to Healing

Transforming Your Pain Through Diet, Exercise, and Lifestyle Changes.

Copyright © 2024 by M K Higgins

All rights reserved. No part of this publication may be reproduced, stored or transmitted in any form or by any means, electronic, mechanical, photocopying, recording, scanning, or otherwise without written permission from the publisher. It is illegal to copy this book, post it to a website, or distribute it by any other means without permission.

M K Higgins asserts the moral right to be identified as the author of this work.

M K Higgins has no responsibility for the persistence or accuracy of URLs for external or third-party Internet Websites referred to in this publication and does not guarantee that any content on such Websites is, or will remain, accurate or appropriate.

Designations used by companies to distinguish their products are often claimed as trademarks. All brand names and product names used in this book and on its cover are trade names, service marks, trademarks and registered trademarks of their respective owners. The publishers and the book are not associated with any product or vendor mentioned in this book. None of the companies referenced within the book have endorsed the book.

First edition

This book was professionally typeset on Reedsy.
Find out more at reedsy.com

Contents

Chapter 1	1
Introduction	1
Chapter 2	3
Managing My Pain	3
Medications	5
Holistic Medicines	8
Empowering Your Healing Journey	10
Other Therapies for Managing Fibromyalgia Pain	11
Not a Single Approach	14
Chapter 3	15
Diet Is Key	15
Finding Your Triggers: What Works and What Doesn't	16
Best Diets for Fibromyalgia: Reducing Inflammation	18
Nutrition and Supplements: Supporting Your Body from Within	19
A Proactive Approach	20
Chapter 4	21
Stretching and Exercise	21
Daily Stretching Your Muscles	22
The Power of Consistency	24
Chapter 5	26
Sleep	26
Environment	27
Regular Exercise	28

Avoid Stimulants	28
Reduce Stress	29
Meditation	29
Listening to Music	30
Magnesium Sulfate Bath Soak	30
Moving Forward: Sleep as a Priority	31
Chapter 6	32
Conclusion	32
Chapter 7	34
Resources	34

Chapter 1

Introduction

Living with fibromyalgia can feel like carrying a weight that no one else can see. It's not just physical pain—it's the fatigue, the brain fog, the tenderness in your body that seems to never go away. The unpredictability can make you feel like you're constantly fighting a battle, but it's a battle that can feel isolated. You're not alone in this, though, and the first step toward managing fibromyalgia is understanding it—and understanding that there is hope for better days ahead.

Fibromyalgia is a chronic condition that affects the way your brain and nervous system process pain signals, amplifying them and turning what should be mild discomfort into excruciating pain. But the pain isn't the whole story. Fibromyalgia impacts many areas of life: sleep patterns, mental clarity, mood, and even the digestive system. It's a condition that varies from person to person, often making it feel like an invisible monster that only you can feel but no one else can see. You might find yourself wondering, Why does this keep happening to me? Why can't I just feel normal again? And those are valid questions. But here's the good news: it's possible to make changes that can lessen the severity of these symptoms and improve your quality of life.

This book is a guide to helping you manage the most common symptoms of fibromyalgia—and to empower you with practical, actionable steps you can start taking right now to feel better. These steps aren't about curing fibromyalgia—unfortunately, there's no magic pill for that. But they are about making choices that can reduce the pain, calm the fatigue, and bring you back to yourself.

Each chapter will focus on a different area of your health and well-being that plays a key role in managing fibromyalgia. From understanding how pain impacts your body, to exploring the healing power of diet, to embracing exercise and sleep as part of your recovery, this book offers you tools to begin feeling better, day by day. The goal isn't perfection. It's progress. Small, sustainable changes that add up to a significant difference over time.

While your fibromyalgia journey is unique to you, remember that there is hope. The changes you make can lead to a life that's more manageable, more joyful, and more centered in your own power. Together, we'll explore the symptoms, challenges, and tools that can help you create your own blueprint. It's time to take the first step. Let's begin this journey to building a blueprint toward healing and empowerment.

Chapter 2

Managing My Pain

Fibromyalgia pain is unlike any other kind of pain. It's persistent, widespread, and often feels like it has no clear cause. For many people, the pain is the hardest part of living with fibromyalgia. It can affect any part of your body at any time, making it feel like a constant companion that never quite leaves. But understanding the nature of this pain is the first step toward managing it.

At its core, fibromyalgia pain is caused by an abnormal response to pain signals in the brain and nervous system. Normally, your body experiences pain as a response to an injury or irritation, and your brain processes it accordingly. But in people with fibromyalgia, the brain and spinal cord process pain signals in an amplified way. What should be mild discomfort can feel like intense, burning, or throbbing pain. This is called "central sensitization"—essentially, your nervous system becomes hyper-sensitive and reacts more strongly than it should to normal stimuli.

This pain can show up in a variety of ways. You might feel deep, aching muscles that never seem to relax, or your joints might feel stiff and tender, as if they're swollen even when they aren't. Some people experience sharp, shooting pains or a sensation of "burning" that radiates from their muscles or joints. It's not uncommon to feel like your whole body is bruised, or like you've been hit by a truck, even after a good night's sleep. The pain can also fluctuate—on some days it may be barely noticeable, and on others, it can be completely debilitating.

For many people with fibromyalgia, pain isn't just a physical symptom—it affects everything. It can influence your mood, your energy, and even your ability to carry out simple daily tasks. You might struggle to get out of bed in the morning, have difficulty sitting or standing for long periods of time, or find that your work and social life are impacted by the unpredictability of flare-ups. Because the pain is chronic, it can also contribute to mental exhaustion, creating a cycle where pain leads to stress, and stress leads to more pain.

The pain of fibromyalgia can also come with a sense of isolation. Since the symptoms are invisible to others, it can be hard for those around you to fully understand the extent of your discomfort. Friends and family may see you looking "fine" on the outside and might not realize that your body is crying out for relief. This can leave you feeling frustrated, misunderstood, and disconnected—compounding the emotional toll of living with chronic pain.

While the pain of fibromyalgia can feel overwhelming at times, it's important to remember that it is manageable. The first step is acknowledging that the pain is not just "in your head," but a real, physiological response. Understanding this can help you feel less defeated by it. There are several effective pain management strategies you can explore to help reduce the intensity and frequency of your pain, and through consistent practice, you can regain a sense of control over your body. In the following sections, we'll look at specific techniques—from mindfulness practices and medication options and alternative treatments—that can help you manage your pain and bring relief when you need it most.

Medications

When it comes to managing fibromyalgia pain, there are a variety of options, and medication is one of them. However, it's important to understand that medication is not the only path, nor is it the right choice for everyone. The decision to take medication is deeply personal, and what works for one person may not work for another. That said, it's crucial to be aware of the different types of medications available, so you can make an informed choice that aligns with your own values, needs, and comfort level.

Medications can be helpful in reducing pain and improving quality of life, but they are just one piece of the puzzle. For some, they offer significant relief and make it possible to engage more fully in daily life. For others, the side effects or concerns about long-term use might outweigh the benefits. The key is finding what feels right for you—and what supports your overall health and well-being.

Pain Relievers - For many people with fibromyalgia, over-the-counter (OTC) pain relievers, such as acetaminophen (Tylenol) or nonsteroidal anti-inflammatory drugs (NSAIDs) like ibuprofen (Advil, Motrin), can provide relief from mild to moderate pain. These medications are often the first step in managing pain, and for some, they are enough to reduce discomfort and help with day-to-day functioning.

However, it's important to keep in mind that these medications are often less effective for the kind of widespread, chronic pain typical of fibromyalgia. Since fibromyalgia pain stems from how the brain processes pain, these pain relievers may not address the root cause of the discomfort. But if you find them helpful, they can be part of a broader strategy for managing pain—just be sure to use them with caution and follow your healthcare provider's advice on dosage and frequency.

Antidepressants - It might sound surprising, but certain antidepressants can help manage fibromyalgia pain. Medications like duloxetine (Cymbalta) and milnacipran (Savella) belong to a class called serotonin-norepinephrine reuptake inhibitors (SNRIs), and they work by balancing brain chemicals that are involved in both pain and mood regulation. For some people, these medications can make a meaningful difference by reducing pain and improving emotional well-being.

Other antidepressants, like tricyclic antidepressants (TCAs), such as amitriptyline and nortriptyline, have also been shown to help with both pain and sleep issues. However, like any medication, they come with potential side effects, such as drowsiness or weight gain, which you should be aware of before making a decision. If you're hesitant about antidepressants, it may help to have an open conversation with your healthcare provider about your concerns and explore whether this option is a good fit for you.

Anti-seizure Medications - Medications like gabapentin (Neurontin) and pregabalin (Lyrica) are often used to manage nerve-related pain, and they can be effective for some people with fibromyalgia. These medications work by calming overactive nerve signals and reducing the pain associated with central sensitization.

While they've been shown to improve pain for many, they may not be suitable for everyone. Common side effects include dizziness, fatigue, and weight gain. If you choose to explore these options, it's important to work closely with your doctor to monitor how you're feeling and adjust the dosage as needed.

Muscle Relaxants - Muscle relaxants, such as cyclobenzaprine (Flexeril), may be recommended for people who experience muscle stiffness and spasms alongside fibromyalgia. These medications can help relieve tension and discomfort in the muscles, which may improve your ability to move more freely. However, they tend to cause drowsiness and may not be ideal for long-term use.

If you're considering a muscle relaxant, it's essential to weigh the benefits against potential side effects and determine if they fit into your overall approach to managing fibromyalgia.

Opioids - **M**edications like oxycodone and hydrocodone— are generally *not* recommended for fibromyalgia. While they may provide temporary relief, they don't address the underlying neurological causes of the pain, and they come with serious risks of dependence and side effects. Most healthcare providers will recommend exploring other, less risky options before considering opioids.

Topical Treatments - For those who prefer a more localized approach to managing pain, topical treatments like creams, gels, or patches can be effective. Products containing ingredients like capsaicin, menthol, or lidocaine can provide targeted relief for specific areas of pain. These treatments are often considered to be low-risk, and many people find them useful when combined with other therapies.

The Decision Is Yours

Ultimately, the choice of whether to use medication—and which medications to try—is yours to make. There is no "one-size-fits-all" solution for fibromyalgia, and what works for one person might not be the right fit for another. If you're unsure about medication, that's completely understandable. Many people with fibromyalgia explore a variety of natural and alternative methods before deciding to turn to pharmaceuticals, and some never choose to use them at all.

What's important is that you're informed and empowered to make decisions that align with your values and your body's needs. Talk to your doctor about your options, ask questions, and don't be afraid to explore all possibilities. Your treatment plan should feel like a partnership between you and your healthcare provider—one that respects your choices and supports your journey toward managing pain in a way that works for you.

Fibromyalgia is complex, and managing its symptoms often requires a combination of approaches. Medications may be one tool in your toolbox, but they don't define your experience. You have the power to explore, experiment, and find what gives you the most relief, whether that's through medication, lifestyle changes, therapies, or a combination of all three.

Holistic Medicines

For many living with fibromyalgia, the idea of managing pain without relying on pharmaceuticals is appealing. Holistic medicines and natural therapies offer an alternative approach that can complement traditional treatments. These options focus on treating the whole person—body, mind, and spirit—and can help alleviate pain and promote overall well-being. While holistic treatments might not provide immediate relief, they can be effective tools in long-term pain management, offering a sense of control and empowerment.

Let's explore a few holistic remedies, including turmeric, an herb that has gained attention for its potential to ease pain.

Turmeric - Turmeric, often praised for its anti-inflammatory properties, contains a compound called curcumin, which has been shown to reduce inflammation and pain. While it is not a cure for fibromyalgia, a study found that turmeric's pain-relieving effects were comparable to over-the-counter pain medications like ibuprofen for some people. For those who prefer a natural remedy, turmeric can be added to your diet or taken as a supplement.

To enhance absorption, it's recommended to consume turmeric with black pepper or fat (such as coconut oil). While research is still ongoing, turmeric may offer a mild yet helpful boost in managing fibromyalgia pain naturally. As with any supplement, be sure to consult your healthcare provider, especially if you are on other medications.

***Magnesium*-** Magnesium is another key mineral that plays a crucial role in managing fibromyalgia pain. Magnesium helps with muscle relaxation, nerve function, and energy production, all of which can help alleviate the muscle stiffness and fatigue associated with fibromyalgia. Many people find relief from their muscle pain by increasing their magnesium intake through food (leafy greens, nuts, seeds) or supplements.

Essential Oils - Aromatherapy using essential oils, such as lavender, peppermint, and eucalyptus, can be a simple yet effective way to manage pain. Lavender is particularly known for its calming properties, which may help reduce stress-related flare-ups, while peppermint and eucalyptus oils have been shown to relieve muscle pain. These oils can be used in a diffuser or applied topically (diluted with a carrier oil) for relief.

Acupuncture - Acupuncture, an ancient practice from Traditional Chinese Medicine, uses thin needles inserted into specific points on the body to restore energy flow and alleviate pain. For fibromyalgia patients, acupuncture may help reduce pain, improve sleep, and reduce fatigue. While results vary, many people find that acupuncture provides lasting relief from muscle and joint pain.

Massage Therapy - Massage is another powerful holistic treatment that can help alleviate muscle pain. By improving circulation and reducing muscle tightness, massage therapy can provide immediate relief for sore muscles. If you suffer from fibromyalgia, regular massage—especially techniques such as Swedish or myofascial release—can help reduce pain and promote relaxation.

Chiropractic Care - Chiropractic care is another holistic treatment option that has been found to benefit individuals with fibromyalgia. Chiropractors focus on the alignment of the spine and musculoskeletal system, using hands-on adjustments to improve spinal function and relieve pain. For fibromyalgia patients, spinal misalignment or tension in the muscles and joints can exacerbate pain and discomfort. Chiropractic adjustments aim to restore proper alignment, improve mobility, and reduce muscle stiffness. Many fibromyalgia patients report experiencing reduced pain and improved range of motion after receiving regular chiropractic care. Additionally, chiropractic treatments may help reduce nerve compression and improve the overall functioning of the nervous system, which can be beneficial given the nervous system's role in amplifying pain in fibromyalgia. If you're considering chiropractic care, it's important to consult with a chiropractor experienced in treating chronic pain conditions like fibromyalgia and work closely with them to develop a treatment plan that supports your overall health and well-being.

Empowering Your Healing Journey

The beauty of holistic medicine is that it offers multiple avenues for pain relief, allowing you to choose what works best for you. Whether you opt for turmeric to reduce inflammation, magnesium for muscle relief, or acupuncture to address deeper imbalances, these treatments offer valuable tools for managing your fibromyalgia symptoms. The key is to listen to your body, be patient, and explore what feels most supportive in your healing journey.

While these options can be incredibly helpful, it's always wise to consult your healthcare provider before starting any new supplement or therapy. Combining natural remedies with other treatments—whether it's medication, physical therapy, or mindfulness practices—can create a well-rounded approach to living with fibromyalgia.

Remember, your path to managing fibromyalgia is uniquely your own, and you have the power to explore, experiment, and discover what makes you feel better—physically, emotionally, and mentally.

Other Therapies for Managing Fibromyalgia Pain

In addition to the more common holistic treatments like magnesium, essential oils, and chiropractic care, there are several other therapies that may help fibromyalgia patients manage their pain and improve their quality of life. These options focus on different aspects of healing, from bodywork to mental health support, and they can be used in combination with other treatments for a more comprehensive approach to managing fibromyalgia symptoms.

Cognitive Behavioral Therapy (CBT) is a form of psychotherapy that focuses on identifying and changing negative thought patterns and behaviors. For people living with fibromyalgia, CBT can be particularly helpful in managing pain and improving emotional well-being. Chronic pain can often lead to feelings of frustration, helplessness, and anxiety, and these emotions can, in turn, exacerbate pain and make it harder to cope. CBT aims to break this cycle by helping individuals reframe their thoughts and develop coping strategies to better manage pain and stress.

Studies have shown that CBT can significantly reduce pain intensity and improve quality of life in fibromyalgia patients. Through CBT, you can learn techniques to manage pain perception, reduce stress, and improve sleep. It is often offered in both individual and group settings, and it can be a valuable complement to other medical or physical treatments.

Biofeedback - is a technique that teaches you how to control physiological functions, such as heart rate, muscle tension, and body temperature, with the goal of reducing stress and managing pain. By using sensors to monitor your body's responses, biofeedback helps you become more aware of how your body reacts to stress and teaches you to control these responses through relaxation techniques, such as deep breathing and muscle relaxation exercises.

For fibromyalgia patients, biofeedback can be an effective way to reduce muscle tension and improve relaxation, which is essential for managing pain. It's often used in combination with other therapies like CBT to address both the mind and body. Biofeedback has been shown to improve sleep quality, reduce anxiety, and help lower the intensity of pain over time.

TENS Therapy - Transcutaneous Electrical Nerve Stimulation (TENS) is a non-invasive treatment that uses low-voltage electrical currents to relieve pain. Small electrodes are placed on the skin near the source of pain, and a mild electrical current is delivered to stimulate the nerves and reduce pain signals. TENS therapy is thought to work by interrupting the pain signals being sent to the brain and promoting the release of endorphins, the body's natural painkillers.

For fibromyalgia patients, TENS can be particularly effective for managing localized pain, such as in the shoulders, back, or knees. It is available through over-the-counter units or can be administered by a physical therapist. While TENS therapy may not completely eliminate pain, many people find it to be a helpful tool for short-term relief and as part of a broader pain management strategy.

Therapeutic Heat and Cold: Simple - Sometimes, the simplest therapies can provide the most relief. Heat and cold treatments, such as heating pads, ice packs, or warm baths, can help alleviate the pain and muscle stiffness that often accompany fibromyalgia. Heat therapy works by increasing blood flow to the affected area, relaxing tense muscles, and soothing aches. Cold therapy, on the other hand, can numb pain and reduce inflammation by constricting blood vessels and limiting swelling.

Many fibromyalgia patients find that alternating between heat and cold provides effective relief, especially for flare-ups. A warm bath with Epsom salts, a heating pad for sore muscles, or a cold pack for joint pain can make a significant difference in managing pain. This is an easy and inexpensive option that can be integrated into your daily routine.

Light Therapy - Fibromyalgia often brings with it sleep disturbances, fatigue, and a disruption of the body's natural circadian rhythms. Light therapy, or bright light exposure, can help reset the body's internal clock and improve sleep quality. This therapy is typically used for conditions like Seasonal Affective Disorder (SAD) but has also been shown to be helpful for people with fibromyalgia who experience significant sleep problems.

Light therapy involves exposure to a light box that mimics natural sunlight, usually for about 20–30 minutes each morning. The light helps regulate the production of melatonin, the hormone that controls sleep, and it can improve mood and energy levels. Regular use of light therapy can help combat the fatigue and low mood that often accompany fibromyalgia.

Mindfulness and Meditation- Mindfulness and meditation are practices that focus on being present in the moment, cultivating awareness of your thoughts, feelings, and bodily sensations. For fibromyalgia patients, mindfulness and meditation techniques can help reduce stress, improve pain tolerance, and promote a sense of calm and control.

Research shows that mindfulness meditation can reduce pain perception and improve overall well-being in people with chronic pain conditions. Practices like deep breathing, body scan meditations, and guided visualization can help you manage stress and better cope with fibromyalgia symptoms. Mindfulness can also help you develop a more compassionate relationship with your body, reducing the mental and emotional toll of chronic pain.

Not a Single Approach

Fibromyalgia treatment is not one specific approach. Finding the right combination of therapies can take time. The therapies mentioned here, from biofeedback and light therapy to TENS and mindfulness practices, are all valuable tools that can help reduce pain, manage stress, and improve your overall quality of life. It's important to remember that no single approach will work for everyone, and you may need to experiment with different methods to find what works best for you.

As always, consult with your healthcare provider before starting any new treatments to ensure they complement your existing care plan. Combining these therapies with proper self-care, lifestyle changes, and a positive mindset can help you regain control over your fibromyalgia and live a more balanced, pain-managed life.

Chapter 3

Diet Is Key

When living with fibromyalgia, managing your diet is one of the most effective ways to influence how your body responds to pain, inflammation, and fatigue. Though fibromyalgia is a complex condition with many contributing factors, your diet plays a key role in either exacerbating or alleviating your symptoms. By paying attention to the foods you eat and the way your body reacts, you can begin to identify dietary patterns that either reduce inflammation or trigger flare-ups.

When it comes to fibromyalgia, each individual's body may react differently to various foods. However, focusing on whole, nutrient-dense foods while cutting out potential triggers can help you manage symptoms and improve overall well-being. The connection between food and fibromyalgia is undeniable, and making dietary changes can offer a significant improvement in your quality of life.

Finding Your Triggers: What Works and What Doesn't

The first step in using diet as a tool to manage fibromyalgia is identifying the foods that may trigger or worsen your symptoms. This process is personal and often involves trial and error, but the benefits of finding your triggers are well worth the effort. Certain foods can contribute to inflammation, digestive issues, and pain, while others may leave you feeling more energized and less fatigued.

Here are some common food triggers that fibromyalgia patients should pay close attention to:

- ***Yeast*** - Yeast, often found in bread, pastries, and processed foods, can be a common trigger for people with fibromyalgia. Yeast overgrowth can lead to digestive discomfort, bloating, and inflammation. If you suspect yeast might be affecting you, consider reducing or eliminating foods that contain yeast, and monitor how your symptoms change.
- ***Nightshades*** - Nightshade vegetables, like tomatoes, potatoes, eggplant, peppers, and tobacco, contain a compound called solanine, which may trigger inflammation and pain in some people with fibromyalgia. While not all individuals with fibromyalgia react to nightshades, eliminating them for a period of time and then reintroducing them can help you determine if they're contributing to your symptoms.
- ***Nitrates*** - Found in processed meats such as bacon, sausage, and deli meats, nitrates can cause inflammation and exacerbate pain. Additionally, nitrates can trigger headaches and digestive distress. If you regularly consume processed meats, you may want to experiment with eliminating them from your diet.
- ***Caffeine*** - Though caffeine may seem like a solution for fatigue, it can actually disrupt sleep patterns and lead to increased tension and

anxiety. Many people with fibromyalgia find that cutting back on or eliminating caffeine from their diet improves their sleep quality and reduces pain sensitivity.

- **Gluten**- For those with fibromyalgia who also have gluten sensitivity or intolerance, gluten can worsen inflammation and contribute to digestive discomfort. If you notice that you feel more fatigued, bloated, or in more pain after consuming gluten, eliminating it may help you feel better. Even if you don't have celiac disease, some people experience gluten sensitivity without realizing it.
- **Dairy** - Dairy products, particularly milk, cheese, and yogurt, can be inflammatory for some people with fibromyalgia. While dairy provides important nutrients, it may also contribute to digestive issues, bloating, and increased pain. If you suspect dairy is a trigger, try eliminating it for a period of time to see if it reduces your symptoms.
- **Chemicals/Dyes in Foods** - Artificial additives, including food dyes, preservatives, and flavor enhancers (like MSG), have been shown to contribute to chronic pain and inflammation. These chemicals can be hidden in many processed foods, snacks, and drinks, so reading labels carefully is essential if you are trying to reduce your intake.
- **Fast Food** - Fast food is often loaded with unhealthy fats, refined sugars, and additives that can trigger inflammation and disrupt your digestion. While it may be convenient, it's also packed with ingredients that can worsen fibromyalgia symptoms. Opting for whole, unprocessed foods whenever possible can make a significant difference in how your body responds to the condition.

Best Diets for Fibromyalgia: Reducing Inflammation

Once you've identified your triggers, the next step is to focus on the foods that will nourish your body and help reduce inflammation. The right diet can have a profound impact on your ability to manage fibromyalgia symptoms.

The Anti-Inflammatory Diet

One of the best dietary approaches for managing fibromyalgia symptoms is the anti-inflammatory diet. This diet emphasizes whole, unprocessed foods that help reduce inflammation and promote healing in the body. It includes foods like:

- Fruits and Vegetables: Rich in antioxidants and anti-inflammatory compounds, fruits like berries and vegetables like spinach, kale, and broccoli can help reduce oxidative stress and fight inflammation.
- Healthy Fats: Omega-3 fatty acids found in fatty fish like salmon, mackerel, and sardines are known for their anti-inflammatory properties. Other healthy fats like those found in olive oil, avocados, and nuts also help reduce inflammation.
- Lean Proteins: Incorporating lean protein sources such as chicken, turkey, and plant-based proteins like lentils and quinoa can provide your body with the nutrients it needs to repair muscles and tissues.
- Whole Grains: Whole grains such as brown rice, quinoa, and oats contain fiber and essential nutrients that support digestive health and help stabilize blood sugar levels.
- Herbs and Spices: Turmeric, ginger, and garlic are well-known for their anti-inflammatory properties. Adding these to your meals can provide both flavor and healing benefits.

The Anti-Inflammatory diet focuses on nutrient-dense, whole foods that can help lower inflammation, reduce pain, and improve your energy levels. By incorporating these foods into your diet and cutting out potential triggers, you can begin to see improvements in how your body feels.

The Mediterranean Diet

The Mediterranean diet is another excellent choice for managing fibromyalgia symptoms. It's rich in fruits, vegetables, whole grains, healthy fats, and lean proteins—particularly from fish and legumes. The Mediterranean diet also emphasizes the importance of herbs and spices like oregano and basil, which contain compounds that help fight inflammation.

Nutrition and Supplements: Supporting Your Body from Within

In addition to adjusting your diet, specific vitamins, minerals, and supplements may help support your body and alleviate fibromyalgia symptoms. While supplements should not replace a healthy diet, they can play a complementary role in managing pain, inflammation, and fatigue.

- Magnesium: Magnesium is essential for muscle function and relaxation. Many fibromyalgia patients are deficient in magnesium, and supplementing with this mineral may help reduce muscle pain, cramps, and spasms. Magnesium-rich foods include leafy greens, nuts, seeds, and whole grains, but taking a magnesium supplement can also be beneficial.
- Vitamin D: Low levels of vitamin D have been associated with increased pain sensitivity and fatigue in people with fibromyalgia.

Supplementing with vitamin D may help improve mood and energy levels, and it plays a crucial role in bone health.
- Omega-3 Fatty Acids: As mentioned earlier, omega-3 fatty acids have powerful anti-inflammatory effects. If you don't regularly consume fatty fish, an omega-3 supplement (like fish oil or algae oil) can help support joint and heart health.
- Probiotics: A healthy gut is crucial for overall well-being, and probiotics can help restore balance to your gut microbiome. This can reduce inflammation and support digestion, which is especially important for fibromyalgia patients.
- Turmeric (Curcumin): Turmeric contains a compound called curcumin, which has potent anti-inflammatory and pain-relieving properties. A curcumin supplement or adding turmeric to your diet can help support pain management, although it's often most effective when combined with black pepper to enhance absorption.
- Coenzyme Q10 (CoQ10): CoQ10 is an antioxidant that helps with energy production at the cellular level. Some studies suggest it can reduce fatigue and improve pain in people with fibromyalgia.

A Proactive Approach

By understanding the role of diet in managing fibromyalgia, you can take a proactive approach to reducing your symptoms and improving your quality of life. Start by identifying your food triggers, then focus on anti-inflammatory foods that support your body's healing process. Consider adding supplements to fill in any nutritional gaps and support your body from the inside out. Through mindful eating and consistent dietary changes, you can find a path to feeling better, with more energy, less pain, and greater overall well-being.

Chapter 4

Stretching and Exercise

Living with fibromyalgia means living with constant discomfort. The pain often feels like it's rooted deep in your muscles, joints, and soft tissues, and the thought of moving—much less exercising—can feel overwhelming. It's not uncommon to want to stay still, to rest, and to avoid activities that might cause more pain. However, the truth is that staying still for too long can make things worse. The muscles in your body, especially the ones affected by fibromyalgia, get tight and stiff, and the fascia—the connective tissue that surrounds your muscles and organs—becomes restricted. Over time, this leads to more pain, more discomfort, and less mobility. The key to breaking this cycle is movement.

Stretching and exercising might feel daunting at first, but it's one of the most important things you can do for your body. The good news is that it doesn't require running marathons or doing high-impact workouts. Instead, it's about taking small, mindful steps to gently stretch and move your body, every day. Over time, this can help reduce pain, improve your flexibility, and increase your overall strength and stamina.

Remember, the goal isn't to push yourself too hard or to adopt a new, rigorous routine. It's about creating a sustainable practice of movement that works for your body and gradually builds over time. Start slow. Be gentle with yourself. And listen to your body. The more you move, the more your body will respond.

Daily Stretching Your Muscles

The muscles in your body can become tight and rigid from fibromyalgia, which can lead to discomfort and reduced range of motion. Stretching is essential for easing this tension and keeping your muscles flexible. A daily stretching routine is one of the simplest and most effective ways to relieve pain, reduce stiffness, and improve mobility.

It doesn't take much to get started—just a few minutes each day can make a significant difference. Focus on gentle, slow stretches that target the major muscle groups, including your neck, shoulders, back, hips, and legs. Try to hold each stretch for about 20-30 seconds, and repeat each one a few times. Stretching can help release tightness in the fascia and muscles, which in turn may reduce pain and discomfort.

It's important to stretch both the large muscle groups (like the quadriceps, hamstrings, and back muscles) as well as the smaller, more specific areas where you tend to feel the most tension (like your neck, shoulders, and calves). Don't force the stretch—move into it slowly and listen to your body. If something feels painful or too intense, back off and try again later.

Walking

Walking is one of the most gentle yet effective forms of exercise you can do when you have fibromyalgia. It's low-impact, it gets your body moving, and it helps with circulation, which can reduce muscle stiffness and improve flexibility. Walking also promotes the release of endorphins—the body's natural painkillers—which can help reduce the perception of pain.

When you first begin, it's important to start slow. Begin with short walks—just five to ten minutes at a time—and gradually increase the duration as your body becomes accustomed to the movement. Pay attention to how your body feels during and after your walks. If you experience a flare-up of symptoms, take a break and allow your body to recover before trying again.

As you continue, aim for at least 20-30 minutes of walking each day. You can split the time into shorter segments if needed. Walking outdoors can also provide the added benefit of fresh air, sunshine, and a change of scenery, which can positively impact your mental well-being.

Yoga

Yoga is a powerful practice that combines stretching, strength, and mindfulness. For fibromyalgia patients, it can help relieve muscle tension, increase flexibility, and reduce stress. Yoga also emphasizes deep breathing, which can be incredibly helpful in managing pain and promoting relaxation. By focusing on both the body and mind, yoga can help break the cycle of stress and pain that often accompanies fibromyalgia.

You don't need to do complicated poses or attend a class to experience the benefits of yoga. Many gentle, restorative yoga practices are specifically designed for those with chronic pain or mobility limitations. Look for yoga classes that focus on flexibility, breathwork, and gentle movements. If you're new to yoga, start with beginner-level sessions or find an online class that emphasizes slow, mindful movements.

•

Tai Chi and Other Gentle Movement Practices

Tai Chi is a low-impact, gentle exercise that has been shown to have significant benefits for people with fibromyalgia. This ancient Chinese practice involves slow, flowing movements and deep breathing. Tai Chi helps improve balance, flexibility, and muscle strength, while also promoting mental clarity and reducing stress. Many people with fibromyalgia find that Tai Chi helps alleviate pain and tension, while also improving overall quality of life.

Other gentle movement practices that can complement your fibromyalgia management. These include Pilates, water aerobics, and Qigong—each of which offers a combination of movement, breathing, and relaxation techniques that can be tailored to your individual needs.

If you're new to Tai Chi, consider attending a beginner class or following along with an online tutorial. Start slowly, focusing on learning the movements rather than pushing yourself to do them perfectly. With regular practice, Tai Chi can help you move with more ease and reduce the physical and emotional strain of fibromyalgia

The Power of Consistency

It's easy to get discouraged when starting a new routine, especially if you've been living with pain for a long time. But the most important thing to remember is that progress comes from consistency, not perfection. Start with small steps, and gradually build your routine as your body allows. You don't need to push yourself too hard—slow, steady movement can have a profound impact on your body over time.

The key to living with fibromyalgia is finding a routine that works for you. Stretching, walking, yoga, and Tai Chi are all accessible, gentle ways to begin moving your body without overwhelming it. By integrating these practices into your daily life, you can begin to break the cycle of pain, reduce tension, and improve your mobility and overall well-being.

Above all, remember to listen to your body. There will be days when

CHAPTER 4

it feels harder to move, and that's okay. Be kind to yourself and take it one day at a time. Each step you take toward movement is a step toward feeling better.

Chapter 5

Sleep

One of the most frustrating aspects of living with fibromyalgia is how it impacts your sleep. We all know how essential sleep is for healing, rest, and overall well-being, but when you have fibromyalgia, getting a good night's sleep can feel like an elusive goal. It's not just the physical pain that keeps you awake—it's the way the condition disrupts the natural rhythm of your brain waves. People with fibromyalgia often experience what's known as "non-restorative sleep," meaning that even though you may sleep for hours, your body doesn't get the deep, rejuvenating rest it needs to repair and recharge. This can leave you feeling exhausted, mentally foggy, and physically drained, no matter how much sleep you get.

What happens in the brain is a bit more complex. Fibromyalgia affects the central nervous system in a way that alters how your brain cycles through the various stages of sleep. In particular, the deeper stages of sleep—when your body repairs and regenerates cells—are often disturbed. The body may enter lighter stages of sleep or wake up more frequently throughout the night. This disruption can leave you feeling like you're not truly resting, even if you've spent hours in bed.

There are several strategies you can implement to help both fall asleep and stay asleep more consistently. The key is to create an environment and routine that signals to your body that it's time to relax and rest. This chapter explores the various approaches you can use to improve the quality of your sleep, from optimizing your sleep environment to managing stress and avoiding the things that disrupt your rest.

Environment

The environment where you sleep plays a huge role in the quality of rest you get. The right environment can help signal to your brain that it's time to unwind and fall into a deep, restorative sleep. But when you live with fibromyalgia, your body is already on high alert due to the pain, so it's important to make your bedroom a haven of calm and relaxation.

Start by making your bedroom as comfortable as possible. Choose bedding that supports your body—memory foam or other supportive mattresses and pillows can help reduce pressure on painful areas. Be mindful of room temperature, as some people with fibromyalgia are sensitive to temperature changes. Try to keep the room cool, but not too cold, and avoid sleeping in a space that's too hot or too stuffy.

Next, think about lighting. Darkness is crucial for signaling your brain that it's time for sleep. If your room has a lot of ambient light, consider blackout curtains or an eye mask. You can also dim the lights an hour or so before bed to help trigger the natural sleep cycle. Your brain needs to know that it's time to rest, and light is one of the strongest signals it uses to determine the time of day.

Finally, consider eliminating noise or distractions that might disrupt your sleep. If you're sensitive to noise, a white noise machine or earplugs can help block out environmental sounds. The goal is to create a peaceful, calming environment where your mind and body can unwind and prepare for rest.

Regular Exercise

We've already discussed the role of movement and exercise in managing fibromyalgia pain, but regular exercise also has a significant impact on sleep quality. Physical activity helps reduce stress, boosts energy levels, and regulates the sleep-wake cycle, making it easier to fall asleep at night.

The key is to find the right type and level of exercise that works for your body. Gentle, low-impact exercises like walking, yoga, and stretching can help prepare your body for sleep by releasing built-up tension and increasing circulation. Aim to finish your exercise routine at least a few hours before bed, as working out too late in the day may make it harder to wind down.

Remember, consistency is more important than intensity. A regular exercise routine, even if it's just a daily walk or stretching session, can help create a healthy rhythm for both your body and your sleep cycle.

Avoid Stimulants

Caffeine is one of the most common culprits when it comes to sleep disturbances, especially if consumed later in the day. As a stimulant, caffeine works by blocking adenosine—a brain chemical that promotes sleep—making it harder for you to fall asleep and stay asleep. Even if you don't typically feel "wired" after drinking coffee or tea, it can still disrupt your body's natural sleep cycle.

Similarly, high sugar intake, especially in the evening, can lead to fluctuations in blood sugar levels, causing energy spikes and crashes that may interfere with your ability to relax at night. If you're struggling with sleep, try limiting your intake of caffeine and sugar, especially in the late afternoon and evening. Opt for herbal teas, like chamomile or valerian root, which can have a calming effect on the body and mind.

Reduce Stress

Stress can exacerbate fibromyalgia pain and make it even harder to sleep. When you're stressed, your body releases hormones like cortisol, which can interfere with your ability to fall into a deep sleep. Managing stress is crucial for improving sleep, and there are several techniques you can use to reduce your stress levels before bed.

One of the most effective ways to manage stress is through relaxation techniques. Deep breathing exercises, progressive muscle relaxation, or guided imagery can help calm your mind and signal to your body that it's time to rest. Consider incorporating a winding-down routine an hour before bed—dim the lights, practice deep breathing, and engage in a calming activity like reading or journaling. This creates a sense of ritual that helps your brain associate these activities with sleep, making it easier to transition into a restful night.

Meditation

For many people with fibromyalgia, the mind can be just as active as the body, making it difficult to fall asleep or stay asleep. Meditation is an excellent tool to quiet the mind and bring a sense of peace and relaxation before bed. Regular meditation practice has been shown to reduce the production of stress hormones and help regulate sleep patterns.

You don't need to meditate for long periods to feel the benefits—just 10-15 minutes of mindful breathing, body scanning, or guided meditation can help shift your mind from a state of hyper-alertness to one of calm. There are many free apps and resources online that provide guided meditations specifically designed for sleep. Experiment with different techniques and find what works best for you.

Listening to Music

Music can be a powerful tool in promoting relaxation and improving sleep. Listening to calming, slow-tempo music before bed has been shown to reduce anxiety, lower heart rate, and enhance feelings of relaxation—all of which help prepare the body for sleep.

Create a playlist of soothing music that you can play each night to signal to your brain that it's time to wind down. Classical music, nature sounds, or ambient instrumental tracks are all great options. The key is to find something that feels peaceful and helps you let go of the day's stress. Music can serve as a gentle transition between the busyness of life and the stillness of sleep.

Magnesium Sulfate Bath Soak

Soaking in a warm **Epsom salt bath** can be a simple and soothing way to help relax your muscles and prepare for sleep. Epsom salts are rich in **magnesium sulfate**, which is thought to be absorbed through the skin to help relax tense muscles, ease pain, and improve sleep quality. Magnesium plays an important role in muscle relaxation and calming the nervous system, both of which are essential for getting a good night's rest.

To use Epsom salts for better sleep, add 1-2 cups of Epsom salts to a warm (but not too hot) bath. Soak for about 10-20 minutes to allow your muscles to relax. This can help ease muscle stiffness, reduce pain, and signal to your body that it's time to unwind and prepare for sleep.

Tip: Be sure to hydrate after your bath, as the warm water can cause fluid loss. Regular use—especially in the evening—can help create a calming nighttime routine that promotes deeper, more restful sleep.

Moving Forward: Sleep as a Priority

Sleep is not a luxury; it's a necessity for both physical and emotional health. For those of us living with fibromyalgia, sleep may feel like a constant struggle, but it is possible to improve the quality of your rest. By creating the right environment, managing your stress, and implementing a soothing pre-sleep routine, you can help calm your body and mind enough to enter a deeper, more restorative sleep.

Remember, there is no one-size-fits-all approach, and it may take time to find the strategies that work best for you. But each small change you make is a step toward getting the rest your body needs to heal, recharge, and face each new day with more energy and resilience.

Chapter 6

Conclusion

Finding Balance and Relief in Your Healing Journey

Living with fibromyalgia is undoubtedly challenging, but throughout this journey, it's important to remember that you are not powerless. The pain, fatigue, and sleep disruptions may feel overwhelming at times, but there are ways to regain control over your body, your health, and your well-being. The blueprint to managing your fibromyalgia isn't about one single solution—it's about a multi-faceted approach that blends self-care, awareness, and proactive strategies. By understanding the unique nature of fibromyalgia pain, learning how to manage it, and adopting lifestyle changes that support your body's needs, you can create a routine that offers relief, enhances your quality of life, and brings you hope for a better tomorrow.

Remember, managing fibromyalgia requires patience, persistence, and a willingness to experiment with different approaches. You may not be able to eliminate all symptoms, but you have the power to make informed choices and build your own blueprint that brings tangible relief. Every small step—whether it's choosing a healthier diet, stretching your muscles, or prioritizing sleep—can help reduce

CHAPTER 6

the impact of fibromyalgia on your life. And while the journey can be unpredictable at times, know that you are not alone. By making mindful, consistent changes, you can create a foundation of well-being and find a rhythm that works for your unique body.

Chapter 7

Resources

Brody, B. (2022, November 29). *Does your diet affect your fibromyalgia?* WebMD. https://www.webmd.com/fibromyalgia/fibromyalgia-and-diet

Exercise and fibromyalgia | HealthLink BC. (n.d.). https://www.healthlinkbc.ca/healthy-eating-physical-activity/conditions/exercise-and-fibromyalgia#:~:text=Mild%20to%20moderate%20exercise%20is,for%20people%20who%20have%20fibromyalgia.

Galan, N., RN. (2018, October 9). *Natural remedies for fibromyalgia.* https://www.medicalnewstoday.com/articles/315393

Liao, S. (2024, February 13). *Fibromyalgia: treatment and medications.* WebMD. https://www.webmd.com/fibromyalgia/medicines-to-treat-fibromyalgia

Pacheco, D., & Pacheco, D. (2023a, December 22). *Fibromyalgia and sleep.* Sleep Foundation. https://www.sleepfoundation.org/physical-health/f

Printed in Great Britain
by Amazon

CHAPTER 7

ibromyalgia-and-sleep

Paultre, K., Cade, W., Hernandez, D., Reynolds, J., Greif, D., & Best, T. M. (2021). Therapeutic effects of turmeric or curcumin extract on pain and function for individuals with knee osteoarthritis: a systematic review. *BMJ Open Sport & Exercise Medicine, 7*(1), e000935. https://doi.org/10.1136/bmjsem-2020-000935

The Fourth Affiliated Hospital of Chengdu University of Traditional Chinese Medicine, Chongqing 400021, China, Department of Rheumatology, Chongqing Hospital of Traditional Chinese Medicine, Chongqing 400021, China, hongqing Key Laboratory of Traditional Chinese Medicine to Prevent and Treat Autoimmune Diseases, Chongqing 400021, China, Department of Rheumatology, Chongqing Hospital of Traditional Chinese Medicine, Chongqing 400021, China, & College of Music, Southwest University, Chongqing 400715, China. (2020). *Music-based interventions to improve fibromyalgia syndrome: A meta-analysis.* Science Direct. Retrieved November 11, 2024, from https://www.sciencedirect.com/science/article/abs/pii/S1550830720301683#:~:text=Conclusions,beneficial%20effects%20of%20music%20therapy.

Chapter 7

Resources

Brody, B. (2022, November 29). *Does your diet affect your fibromyalgia?* WebMD. https://www.webmd.com/fibromyalgia/fibromyalgia-and-diet

Exercise and fibromyalgia | HealthLink BC. (n.d.). https://www.healthlinkbc.ca/healthy-eating-physical-activity/conditions/exercise-and-fibromyalgia#:~:text=Mild%20to%20moderate%20exercise%20is,for%20people%20who%20have%20fibromyalgia.

Galan, N., RN. (2018, October 9). *Natural remedies for fibromyalgia.* https://www.medicalnewstoday.com/articles/315393

Liao, S. (2024, February 13). *Fibromyalgia: treatment and medications.* WebMD. https://www.webmd.com/fibromyalgia/medicines-to-treat-fibromyalgia

Pacheco, D., & Pacheco, D. (2023a, December 22). *Fibromyalgia and sleep.* Sleep Foundation. https://www.sleepfoundation.org/physical-health/f

CHAPTER 6

the impact of fibromyalgia on your life. And while the journey can be unpredictable at times, know that you are not alone. By making mindful, consistent changes, you can create a foundation of well-being and find a rhythm that works for your unique body.

Chapter 6

Conclusion

Finding Balance and Relief in Your Healing Journey
Living with fibromyalgia is undoubtedly challenging, but throughout this journey, it's important to remember that you are not powerless. The pain, fatigue, and sleep disruptions may feel overwhelming at times, but there are ways to regain control over your body, your health, and your well-being. The blueprint to managing your fibromyalgia isn't about one single solution—it's about a multi-faceted approach that blends self-care, awareness, and proactive strategies. By understanding the unique nature of fibromyalgia pain, learning how to manage it, and adopting lifestyle changes that support your body's needs, you can create a routine that offers relief, enhances your quality of life, and brings you hope for a better tomorrow.

Remember, managing fibromyalgia requires patience, persistence, and a willingness to experiment with different approaches. You may not be able to eliminate all symptoms, but you have the power to make informed choices and build your own blueprint that brings tangible relief. Every small step—whether it's choosing a healthier diet, stretching your muscles, or prioritizing sleep—can help reduce

To use Epsom salts for better sleep, add 1-2 cups of Epsom salts to a warm (but not too hot) bath. Soak for about 10-20 minutes to allow your muscles to relax. This can help ease muscle stiffness, reduce pain, and signal to your body that it's time to unwind and prepare for sleep.

Tip: Be sure to hydrate after your bath, as the warm water can cause fluid loss. Regular use—especially in the evening—can help create a calming nighttime routine that promotes deeper, more restful sleep.

Moving Forward: Sleep as a Priority

Sleep is not a luxury; it's a necessity for both physical and emotional health. For those of us living with fibromyalgia, sleep may feel like a constant struggle, but it is possible to improve the quality of your rest. By creating the right environment, managing your stress, and implementing a soothing pre-sleep routine, you can help calm your body and mind enough to enter a deeper, more restorative sleep.

Remember, there is no one-size-fits-all approach, and it may take time to find the strategies that work best for you. But each small change you make is a step toward getting the rest your body needs to heal, recharge, and face each new day with more energy and resilience.

You don't need to meditate for long periods to feel the benefits—just 10-15 minutes of mindful breathing, body scanning, or guided meditation can help shift your mind from a state of hyper-alertness to one of calm. There are many free apps and resources online that provide guided meditations specifically designed for sleep. Experiment with different techniques and find what works best for you.

Listening to Music

Music can be a powerful tool in promoting relaxation and improving sleep. Listening to calming, slow-tempo music before bed has been shown to reduce anxiety, lower heart rate, and enhance feelings of relaxation—all of which help prepare the body for sleep.

Create a playlist of soothing music that you can play each night to signal to your brain that it's time to wind down. Classical music, nature sounds, or ambient instrumental tracks are all great options. The key is to find something that feels peaceful and helps you let go of the day's stress. Music can serve as a gentle transition between the busyness of life and the stillness of sleep.

Magnesium Sulfate Bath Soak

Soaking in a warm **Epsom salt bath** can be a simple and soothing way to help relax your muscles and prepare for sleep. Epsom salts are rich in **magnesium sulfate**, which is thought to be absorbed through the skin to help relax tense muscles, ease pain, and improve sleep quality. Magnesium plays an important role in muscle relaxation and calming the nervous system, both of which are essential for getting a good night's rest.

that may interfere with your ability to relax at night. If you're struggling with sleep, try limiting your intake of caffeine and sugar, especially in the late afternoon and evening. Opt for herbal teas, like chamomile or valerian root, which can have a calming effect on the body and mind.

Reduce Stress

Stress can exacerbate fibromyalgia pain and make it even harder to sleep. When you're stressed, your body releases hormones like cortisol, which can interfere with your ability to fall into a deep sleep. Managing stress is crucial for improving sleep, and there are several techniques you can use to reduce your stress levels before bed.

One of the most effective ways to manage stress is through relaxation techniques. Deep breathing exercises, progressive muscle relaxation, or guided imagery can help calm your mind and signal to your body that it's time to rest. Consider incorporating a winding-down routine an hour before bed—dim the lights, practice deep breathing, and engage in a calming activity like reading or journaling. This creates a sense of ritual that helps your brain associate these activities with sleep, making it easier to transition into a restful night.

Meditation

For many people with fibromyalgia, the mind can be just as active as the body, making it difficult to fall asleep or stay asleep. Meditation is an excellent tool to quiet the mind and bring a sense of peace and relaxation before bed. Regular meditation practice has been shown to reduce the production of stress hormones and help regulate sleep patterns.

and prepare for rest.

Regular Exercise

We've already discussed the role of movement and exercise in managing fibromyalgia pain, but regular exercise also has a significant impact on sleep quality. Physical activity helps reduce stress, boosts energy levels, and regulates the sleep-wake cycle, making it easier to fall asleep at night.

The key is to find the right type and level of exercise that works for your body. Gentle, low-impact exercises like walking, yoga, and stretching can help prepare your body for sleep by releasing built-up tension and increasing circulation. Aim to finish your exercise routine at least a few hours before bed, as working out too late in the day may make it harder to wind down.

Remember, consistency is more important than intensity. A regular exercise routine, even if it's just a daily walk or stretching session, can help create a healthy rhythm for both your body and your sleep cycle.

Avoid Stimulants

Caffeine is one of the most common culprits when it comes to sleep disturbances, especially if consumed later in the day. As a stimulant, caffeine works by blocking adenosine—a brain chemical that promotes sleep—making it harder for you to fall asleep and stay asleep. Even if you don't typically feel "wired" after drinking coffee or tea, it can still disrupt your body's natural sleep cycle.

Similarly, high sugar intake, especially in the evening, can lead to fluctuations in blood sugar levels, causing energy spikes and crashes and stay asleep more consistently. The key is to create an environment and routine that signals to your body that it's time to relax and rest. This chapter explores the various approaches you can use to improve the quality of your sleep, from optimizing your sleep environment to managing stress and avoiding the things that disrupt your rest.

Environment

The environment where you sleep plays a huge role in the quality of rest you get. The right environment can help signal to your brain that it's time to unwind and fall into a deep, restorative sleep. But when you live with fibromyalgia, your body is already on high alert due to the pain, so it's important to make your bedroom a haven of calm and relaxation.

Start by making your bedroom as comfortable as possible. Choose bedding that supports your body—memory foam or other supportive mattresses and pillows can help reduce pressure on painful areas. Be mindful of room temperature, as some people with fibromyalgia are sensitive to temperature changes. Try to keep the room cool, but not too cold, and avoid sleeping in a space that's too hot or too stuffy.

Next, think about lighting. Darkness is crucial for signaling your brain that it's time for sleep. If your room has a lot of ambient light, consider blackout curtains or an eye mask. You can also dim the lights an hour or so before bed to help trigger the natural sleep cycle. Your brain needs to know that it's time to rest, and light is one of the strongest signals it uses to determine the time of day.

Finally, consider eliminating noise or distractions that might disrupt your sleep. If you're sensitive to noise, a white noise machine or earplugs can help block out environmental sounds. The goal is to create a peaceful, calming environment where your mind and body can unwind

Chapter 5

Sleep

One of the most frustrating aspects of living with fibromyalgia is how it impacts your sleep. We all know how essential sleep is for healing, rest, and overall well-being, but when you have fibromyalgia, getting a good night's sleep can feel like an elusive goal. It's not just the physical pain that keeps you awake—it's the way the condition disrupts the natural rhythm of your brain waves. People with fibromyalgia often experience what's known as "non-restorative sleep," meaning that even though you may sleep for hours, your body doesn't get the deep, rejuvenating rest it needs to repair and recharge. This can leave you feeling exhausted, mentally foggy, and physically drained, no matter how much sleep you get.

What happens in the brain is a bit more complex. Fibromyalgia affects the central nervous system in a way that alters how your brain cycles through the various stages of sleep. In particular, the deeper stages of sleep—when your body repairs and regenerates cells—are often disturbed. The body may enter lighter stages of sleep or wake up more frequently throughout the night. This disruption can leave you feeling like you're not truly resting, even if you've spent hours in bed.

There are several strategies you can implement to help both fall asleep it feels harder to move, and that's okay. Be kind to yourself and take it one day at a time. Each step you take toward movement is a step toward feeling better.

have significant benefits for people with fibromyalgia. This ancient Chinese practice involves slow, flowing movements and deep breathing. Tai Chi helps improve balance, flexibility, and muscle strength, while also promoting mental clarity and reducing stress. Many people with fibromyalgia find that Tai Chi helps alleviate pain and tension, while also improving overall quality of life.

Other gentle movement practices that can complement your fibromyalgia management. These include Pilates, water aerobics, and Qigong—each of which offers a combination of movement, breathing, and relaxation techniques that can be tailored to your individual needs.

If you're new to Tai Chi, consider attending a beginner class or following along with an online tutorial. Start slowly, focusing on learning the movements rather than pushing yourself to do them perfectly. With regular practice, Tai Chi can help you move with more ease and reduce the physical and emotional strain of fibromyalgia

The Power of Consistency

It's easy to get discouraged when starting a new routine, especially if you've been living with pain for a long time. But the most important thing to remember is that progress comes from consistency, not perfection. Start with small steps, and gradually build your routine as your body allows. You don't need to push yourself too hard—slow, steady movement can have a profound impact on your body over time.

The key to living with fibromyalgia is finding a routine that works for you. Stretching, walking, yoga, and Tai Chi are all accessible, gentle ways to begin moving your body without overwhelming it. By integrating these practices into your daily life, you can begin to break the cycle of pain, reduce tension, and improve your mobility and overall well-being.

Above all, remember to listen to your body. There will be days when perception of pain.

When you first begin, it's important to start slow. Begin with short walks—just five to ten minutes at a time—and gradually increase the duration as your body becomes accustomed to the movement. Pay attention to how your body feels during and after your walks. If you experience a flare-up of symptoms, take a break and allow your body to recover before trying again.

As you continue, aim for at least 20-30 minutes of walking each day. You can split the time into shorter segments if needed. Walking outdoors can also provide the added benefit of fresh air, sunshine, and a change of scenery, which can positively impact your mental well-being.

Yoga

Yoga is a powerful practice that combines stretching, strength, and mindfulness. For fibromyalgia patients, it can help relieve muscle tension, increase flexibility, and reduce stress. Yoga also emphasizes deep breathing, which can be incredibly helpful in managing pain and promoting relaxation. By focusing on both the body and mind, yoga can help break the cycle of stress and pain that often accompanies fibromyalgia.

You don't need to do complicated poses or attend a class to experience the benefits of yoga. Many gentle, restorative yoga practices are specifically designed for those with chronic pain or mobility limitations. Look for yoga classes that focus on flexibility, breathwork, and gentle movements. If you're new to yoga, start with beginner-level sessions or find an online class that emphasizes slow, mindful movements.

-

Tai Chi and Other Gentle Movement Practices

Tai Chi is a low-impact, gentle exercise that has been shown to that works for your body and gradually builds over time. Start slow. Be gentle with yourself. And listen to your body. The more you move, the more your body will respond.

Daily Stretching Your Muscles

The muscles in your body can become tight and rigid from fibromyalgia, which can lead to discomfort and reduced range of motion. Stretching is essential for easing this tension and keeping your muscles flexible. A daily stretching routine is one of the simplest and most effective ways to relieve pain, reduce stiffness, and improve mobility.

It doesn't take much to get started—just a few minutes each day can make a significant difference. Focus on gentle, slow stretches that target the major muscle groups, including your neck, shoulders, back, hips, and legs. Try to hold each stretch for about 20-30 seconds, and repeat each one a few times. Stretching can help release tightness in the fascia and muscles, which in turn may reduce pain and discomfort.

It's important to stretch both the large muscle groups (like the quadriceps, hamstrings, and back muscles) as well as the smaller, more specific areas where you tend to feel the most tension (like your neck, shoulders, and calves). Don't force the stretch—move into it slowly and listen to your body. If something feels painful or too intense, back off and try again later.

Walking

Walking is one of the most gentle yet effective forms of exercise you can do when you have fibromyalgia. It's low-impact, it gets your body moving, and it helps with circulation, which can reduce muscle stiffness and improve flexibility. Walking also promotes the release of endorphins—the body's natural painkillers—which can help reduce the

Chapter 4

Stretching and Exercise

Living with fibromyalgia means living with constant discomfort. The pain often feels like it's rooted deep in your muscles, joints, and soft tissues, and the thought of moving—much less exercising—can feel overwhelming. It's not uncommon to want to stay still, to rest, and to avoid activities that might cause more pain. However, the truth is that staying still for too long can make things worse. The muscles in your body, especially the ones affected by fibromyalgia, get tight and stiff, and the fascia—the connective tissue that surrounds your muscles and organs—becomes restricted. Over time, this leads to more pain, more discomfort, and less mobility. The key to breaking this cycle is movement.

Stretching and exercising might feel daunting at first, but it's one of the most important things you can do for your body. The good news is that it doesn't require running marathons or doing high-impact workouts. Instead, it's about taking small, mindful steps to gently stretch and move your body, every day. Over time, this can help reduce pain, improve your flexibility, and increase your overall strength and stamina.

Remember, the goal isn't to push yourself too hard or to adopt a new, rigorous routine. It's about creating a sustainable practice of movement

Supplementing with vitamin D may help improve mood and energy levels, and it plays a crucial role in bone health.
- Omega-3 Fatty Acids: As mentioned earlier, omega-3 fatty acids have powerful anti-inflammatory effects. If you don't regularly consume fatty fish, an omega-3 supplement (like fish oil or algae oil) can help support joint and heart health.
- Probiotics: A healthy gut is crucial for overall well-being, and probiotics can help restore balance to your gut microbiome. This can reduce inflammation and support digestion, which is especially important for fibromyalgia patients.
- Turmeric (Curcumin): Turmeric contains a compound called curcumin, which has potent anti-inflammatory and pain-relieving properties. A curcumin supplement or adding turmeric to your diet can help support pain management, although it's often most effective when combined with black pepper to enhance absorption.
- Coenzyme Q10 (CoQ10): CoQ10 is an antioxidant that helps with energy production at the cellular level. Some studies suggest it can reduce fatigue and improve pain in people with fibromyalgia.

A Proactive Approach

By understanding the role of diet in managing fibromyalgia, you can take a proactive approach to reducing your symptoms and improving your quality of life. Start by identifying your food triggers, then focus on anti-inflammatory foods that support your body's healing process. Consider adding supplements to fill in any nutritional gaps and support your body from the inside out. Through mindful eating and consistent dietary changes, you can find a path to feeling better, with more energy, less pain, and greater overall well-being.

that can help lower inflammation, reduce pain, and improve your energy levels. By incorporating these foods into your diet and cutting out potential triggers, you can begin to see improvements in how your body feels.

The Mediterranean Diet

The Mediterranean diet is another excellent choice for managing fibromyalgia symptoms. It's rich in fruits, vegetables, whole grains, healthy fats, and lean proteins—particularly from fish and legumes. The Mediterranean diet also emphasizes the importance of herbs and spices like oregano and basil, which contain compounds that help fight inflammation.

Nutrition and Supplements: Supporting Your Body from Within

In addition to adjusting your diet, specific vitamins, minerals, and supplements may help support your body and alleviate fibromyalgia symptoms. While supplements should not replace a healthy diet, they can play a complementary role in managing pain, inflammation, and fatigue.

- Magnesium: Magnesium is essential for muscle function and relaxation. Many fibromyalgia patients are deficient in magnesium, and supplementing with this mineral may help reduce muscle pain, cramps, and spasms. Magnesium-rich foods include leafy greens, nuts, seeds, and whole grains, but taking a magnesium supplement can also be beneficial.
- Vitamin D: Low levels of vitamin D have been associated with increased pain sensitivity and fatigue in people with fibromyalgia.

Best Diets for Fibromyalgia: Reducing Inflammation

Once you've identified your triggers, the next step is to focus on the foods that will nourish your body and help reduce inflammation. The right diet can have a profound impact on your ability to manage fibromyalgia symptoms.

The Anti-Inflammatory Diet

One of the best dietary approaches for managing fibromyalgia symptoms is the anti-inflammatory diet. This diet emphasizes whole, unprocessed foods that help reduce inflammation and promote healing in the body. It includes foods like:

- Fruits and Vegetables: Rich in antioxidants and anti-inflammatory compounds, fruits like berries and vegetables like spinach, kale, and broccoli can help reduce oxidative stress and fight inflammation.
- Healthy Fats: Omega-3 fatty acids found in fatty fish like salmon, mackerel, and sardines are known for their anti-inflammatory properties. Other healthy fats like those found in olive oil, avocados, and nuts also help reduce inflammation.
- Lean Proteins: Incorporating lean protein sources such as chicken, turkey, and plant-based proteins like lentils and quinoa can provide your body with the nutrients it needs to repair muscles and tissues.
- Whole Grains: Whole grains such as brown rice, quinoa, and oats contain fiber and essential nutrients that support digestive health and help stabilize blood sugar levels.
- Herbs and Spices: Turmeric, ginger, and garlic are well-known for their anti-inflammatory properties. Adding these to your meals can provide both flavor and healing benefits.

The Anti-Inflammatory diet focuses on nutrient-dense, whole foods anxiety. Many people with fibromyalgia find that cutting back on or eliminating caffeine from their diet improves their sleep quality and reduces pain sensitivity.

- *Gluten*- For those with fibromyalgia who also have gluten sensitivity or intolerance, gluten can worsen inflammation and contribute to digestive discomfort. If you notice that you feel more fatigued, bloated, or in more pain after consuming gluten, eliminating it may help you feel better. Even if you don't have celiac disease, some people experience gluten sensitivity without realizing it.
- *Dairy* - Dairy products, particularly milk, cheese, and yogurt, can be inflammatory for some people with fibromyalgia. While dairy provides important nutrients, it may also contribute to digestive issues, bloating, and increased pain. If you suspect dairy is a trigger, try eliminating it for a period of time to see if it reduces your symptoms.
- *Chemicals/Dyes in Foods* - Artificial additives, including food dyes, preservatives, and flavor enhancers (like MSG), have been shown to contribute to chronic pain and inflammation. These chemicals can be hidden in many processed foods, snacks, and drinks, so reading labels carefully is essential if you are trying to reduce your intake.
- *Fast Food* - Fast food is often loaded with unhealthy fats, refined sugars, and additives that can trigger inflammation and disrupt your digestion. While it may be convenient, it's also packed with ingredients that can worsen fibromyalgia symptoms. Opting for whole, unprocessed foods whenever possible can make a significant difference in how your body responds to the condition.

Finding Your Triggers: What Works and What Doesn't

The first step in using diet as a tool to manage fibromyalgia is identifying the foods that may trigger or worsen your symptoms. This process is personal and often involves trial and error, but the benefits of finding your triggers are well worth the effort. Certain foods can contribute to inflammation, digestive issues, and pain, while others may leave you feeling more energized and less fatigued.

Here are some common food triggers that fibromyalgia patients should pay close attention to:

- **Yeast**- Yeast, often found in bread, pastries, and processed foods, can be a common trigger for people with fibromyalgia. Yeast overgrowth can lead to digestive discomfort, bloating, and inflammation. If you suspect yeast might be affecting you, consider reducing or eliminating foods that contain yeast, and monitor how your symptoms change.
- **Nightshades** - Nightshade vegetables, like tomatoes, potatoes, eggplant, peppers, and tobacco, contain a compound called solanine, which may trigger inflammation and pain in some people with fibromyalgia. While not all individuals with fibromyalgia react to nightshades, eliminating them for a period of time and then reintroducing them can help you determine if they're contributing to your symptoms.
- **Nitrates** - Found in processed meats such as bacon, sausage, and deli meats, nitrates can cause inflammation and exacerbate pain. Additionally, nitrates can trigger headaches and digestive distress. If you regularly consume processed meats, you may want to experiment with eliminating them from your diet.
- **Caffeine** - Though caffeine may seem like a solution for fatigue, it can actually disrupt sleep patterns and lead to increased tension and

Chapter 3

Diet Is Key

When living with fibromyalgia, managing your diet is one of the most effective ways to influence how your body responds to pain, inflammation, and fatigue. Though fibromyalgia is a complex condition with many contributing factors, your diet plays a key role in either exacerbating or alleviating your symptoms. By paying attention to the foods you eat and the way your body reacts, you can begin to identify dietary patterns that either reduce inflammation or trigger flare-ups.

When it comes to fibromyalgia, each individual's body may react differently to various foods. However, focusing on whole, nutrient-dense foods while cutting out potential triggers can help you manage symptoms and improve overall well-being. The connection between food and fibromyalgia is undeniable, and making dietary changes can offer a significant improvement in your quality of life.

Mindfulness and Meditation- Mindfulness and meditation are practices that focus on being present in the moment, cultivating awareness of your thoughts, feelings, and bodily sensations. For fibromyalgia patients, mindfulness and meditation techniques can help reduce stress, improve pain tolerance, and promote a sense of calm and control.

Research shows that mindfulness meditation can reduce pain perception and improve overall well-being in people with chronic pain conditions. Practices like deep breathing, body scan meditations, and guided visualization can help you manage stress and better cope with fibromyalgia symptoms. Mindfulness can also help you develop a more compassionate relationship with your body, reducing the mental and emotional toll of chronic pain.

Not a Single Approach

Fibromyalgia treatment is not one specific approach. Finding the right combination of therapies can take time. The therapies mentioned here, from biofeedback and light therapy to TENS and mindfulness practices, are all valuable tools that can help reduce pain, manage stress, and improve your overall quality of life. It's important to remember that no single approach will work for everyone, and you may need to experiment with different methods to find what works best for you.

As always, consult with your healthcare provider before starting any new treatments to ensure they complement your existing care plan. Combining these therapies with proper self-care, lifestyle changes, and a positive mindset can help you regain control over your fibromyalgia and live a more balanced, pain-managed life.

physical therapist. While TENS therapy may not completely eliminate pain, many people find it to be a helpful tool for short-term relief and as part of a broader pain management strategy.

Therapeutic Heat and Cold: Simple - Sometimes, the simplest therapies can provide the most relief. Heat and cold treatments, such as heating pads, ice packs, or warm baths, can help alleviate the pain and muscle stiffness that often accompany fibromyalgia. Heat therapy works by increasing blood flow to the affected area, relaxing tense muscles, and soothing aches. Cold therapy, on the other hand, can numb pain and reduce inflammation by constricting blood vessels and limiting swelling.

Many fibromyalgia patients find that alternating between heat and cold provides effective relief, especially for flare-ups. A warm bath with Epsom salts, a heating pad for sore muscles, or a cold pack for joint pain can make a significant difference in managing pain. This is an easy and inexpensive option that can be integrated into your daily routine.

Light Therapy - Fibromyalgia often brings with it sleep disturbances, fatigue, and a disruption of the body's natural circadian rhythms. Light therapy, or bright light exposure, can help reset the body's internal clock and improve sleep quality. This therapy is typically used for conditions like Seasonal Affective Disorder (SAD) but has also been shown to be helpful for people with fibromyalgia who experience significant sleep problems.

Light therapy involves exposure to a light box that mimics natural sunlight, usually for about 20–30 minutes each morning. The light helps regulate the production of melatonin, the hormone that controls sleep, and it can improve mood and energy levels. Regular use of light therapy can help combat the fatigue and low mood that often accompany fibromyalgia.

Studies have shown that CBT can significantly reduce pain intensity and improve quality of life in fibromyalgia patients. Through CBT, you can learn techniques to manage pain perception, reduce stress, and improve sleep. It is often offered in both individual and group settings, and it can be a valuable complement to other medical or physical treatments.

Biofeedback - is a technique that teaches you how to control physiological functions, such as heart rate, muscle tension, and body temperature, with the goal of reducing stress and managing pain. By using sensors to monitor your body's responses, biofeedback helps you become more aware of how your body reacts to stress and teaches you to control these responses through relaxation techniques, such as deep breathing and muscle relaxation exercises.

For fibromyalgia patients, biofeedback can be an effective way to reduce muscle tension and improve relaxation, which is essential for managing pain. It's often used in combination with other therapies like CBT to address both the mind and body. Biofeedback has been shown to improve sleep quality, reduce anxiety, and help lower the intensity of pain over time.

TENS Therapy - Transcutaneous Electrical Nerve Stimulation (TENS) is a non-invasive treatment that uses low-voltage electrical currents to relieve pain. Small electrodes are placed on the skin near the source of pain, and a mild electrical current is delivered to stimulate the nerves and reduce pain signals. TENS therapy is thought to work by interrupting the pain signals being sent to the brain and promoting the release of endorphins, the body's natural painkillers.

For fibromyalgia patients, TENS can be particularly effective for managing localized pain, such as in the shoulders, back, or knees. It is available through over-the-counter units or can be administered by a offer valuable tools for managing your fibromyalgia symptoms. The key is to listen to your body, be patient, and explore what feels most supportive in your healing journey.

While these options can be incredibly helpful, it's always wise to consult your healthcare provider before starting any new supplement or therapy. Combining natural remedies with other treatments—whether it's medication, physical therapy, or mindfulness practices—can create a well-rounded approach to living with fibromyalgia.

Remember, your path to managing fibromyalgia is uniquely your own, and you have the power to explore, experiment, and discover what makes you feel better—physically, emotionally, and mentally.

Other Therapies for Managing Fibromyalgia Pain

In addition to the more common holistic treatments like magnesium, essential oils, and chiropractic care, there are several other therapies that may help fibromyalgia patients manage their pain and improve their quality of life. These options focus on different aspects of healing, from bodywork to mental health support, and they can be used in combination with other treatments for a more comprehensive approach to managing fibromyalgia symptoms.

Cognitive Behavioral Therapy (CBT) is a form of psychotherapy that focuses on identifying and changing negative thought patterns and behaviors. For people living with fibromyalgia, CBT can be particularly helpful in managing pain and improving emotional well-being. Chronic pain can often lead to feelings of frustration, helplessness, and anxiety, and these emotions can, in turn, exacerbate pain and make it harder to cope. CBT aims to break this cycle by helping individuals reframe their thoughts and develop coping strategies to better manage pain and stress.

can help alleviate muscle pain. By improving circulation and reducing muscle tightness, massage therapy can provide immediate relief for sore muscles. If you suffer from fibromyalgia, regular massage—especially techniques such as Swedish or myofascial release—can help reduce pain and promote relaxation.

Chiropractic Care - Chiropractic care is another holistic treatment option that has been found to benefit individuals with fibromyalgia. Chiropractors focus on the alignment of the spine and musculoskeletal system, using hands-on adjustments to improve spinal function and relieve pain. For fibromyalgia patients, spinal misalignment or tension in the muscles and joints can exacerbate pain and discomfort. Chiropractic adjustments aim to restore proper alignment, improve mobility, and reduce muscle stiffness. Many fibromyalgia patients report experiencing reduced pain and improved range of motion after receiving regular chiropractic care. Additionally, chiropractic treatments may help reduce nerve compression and improve the overall functioning of the nervous system, which can be beneficial given the nervous system's role in amplifying pain in fibromyalgia. If you're considering chiropractic care, it's important to consult with a chiropractor experienced in treating chronic pain conditions like fibromyalgia and work closely with them to develop a treatment plan that supports your overall health and well-being.

Empowering Your Healing Journey

The beauty of holistic medicine is that it offers multiple avenues for pain relief, allowing you to choose what works best for you. Whether you opt for turmeric to reduce inflammation, magnesium for muscle relief, or acupuncture to address deeper imbalances, these treatments who prefer a natural remedy, turmeric can be added to your diet or taken as a supplement.

To enhance absorption, it's recommended to consume turmeric with black pepper or fat (such as coconut oil). While research is still ongoing, turmeric may offer a mild yet helpful boost in managing fibromyalgia pain naturally. As with any supplement, be sure to consult your healthcare provider, especially if you are on other medications.

Magnesium- Magnesium is another key mineral that plays a crucial role in managing fibromyalgia pain. Magnesium helps with muscle relaxation, nerve function, and energy production, all of which can help alleviate the muscle stiffness and fatigue associated with fibromyalgia. Many people find relief from their muscle pain by increasing their magnesium intake through food (leafy greens, nuts, seeds) or supplements.

Essential Oils - Aromatherapy using essential oils, such as lavender, peppermint, and eucalyptus, can be a simple yet effective way to manage pain. Lavender is particularly known for its calming properties, which may help reduce stress-related flare-ups, while peppermint and eucalyptus oils have been shown to relieve muscle pain. These oils can be used in a diffuser or applied topically (diluted with a carrier oil) for relief.

Acupuncture - Acupuncture, an ancient practice from Traditional Chinese Medicine, uses thin needles inserted into specific points on the body to restore energy flow and alleviate pain. For fibromyalgia patients, acupuncture may help reduce pain, improve sleep, and reduce fatigue. While results vary, many people find that acupuncture provides lasting relief from muscle and joint pain.

Massage Therapy - Massage is another powerful holistic treatment that all possibilities. Your treatment plan should feel like a partnership between you and your healthcare provider—one that respects your choices and supports your journey toward managing pain in a way that works for you.

Fibromyalgia is complex, and managing its symptoms often requires a combination of approaches. Medications may be one tool in your toolbox, but they don't define your experience. You have the power to explore, experiment, and find what gives you the most relief, whether that's through medication, lifestyle changes, therapies, or a combination of all three.

Holistic Medicines

For many living with fibromyalgia, the idea of managing pain without relying on pharmaceuticals is appealing. Holistic medicines and natural therapies offer an alternative approach that can complement traditional treatments. These options focus on treating the whole person—body, mind, and spirit—and can help alleviate pain and promote overall well-being. While holistic treatments might not provide immediate relief, they can be effective tools in long-term pain management, offering a sense of control and empowerment.

Let's explore a few holistic remedies, including turmeric, an herb that has gained attention for its potential to ease pain.

Turmeric - Turmeric, often praised for its anti-inflammatory properties, contains a compound called curcumin, which has been shown to reduce inflammation and pain. While it is not a cure for fibromyalgia, a study found that turmeric's pain-relieving effects were comparable to over-the-counter pain medications like ibuprofen for some people. For those to move more freely. However, they tend to cause drowsiness and may not be ideal for long-term use.

If you're considering a muscle relaxant, it's essential to weigh the benefits against potential side effects and determine if they fit into your overall approach to managing fibromyalgia.

Opioids - Medications like oxycodone and hydrocodone— are generally *not* recommended for fibromyalgia. While they may provide temporary relief, they don't address the underlying neurological causes of the pain, and they come with serious risks of dependence and side effects. Most healthcare providers will recommend exploring other, less risky options before considering opioids.

Topical Treatments - For those who prefer a more localized approach to managing pain, topical treatments like creams, gels, or patches can be effective. Products containing ingredients like capsaicin, menthol, or lidocaine can provide targeted relief for specific areas of pain. These treatments are often considered to be low-risk, and many people find them useful when combined with other therapies.

The Decision Is Yours

Ultimately, the choice of whether to use medication—and which medications to try—is yours to make. There is no "one-size-fits-all" solution for fibromyalgia, and what works for one person might not be the right fit for another. If you're unsure about medication, that's completely understandable. Many people with fibromyalgia explore a variety of natural and alternative methods before deciding to turn to pharmaceuticals, and some never choose to use them at all.

What's important is that you're informed and empowered to make decisions that align with your values and your body's needs. Talk to your doctor about your options, ask questions, and don't be afraid to explore

Antidepressants - It might sound surprising, but certain antidepressants can help manage fibromyalgia pain. Medications like duloxetine (Cymbalta) and milnacipran (Savella) belong to a class called serotonin-norepinephrine reuptake inhibitors (SNRIs), and they work by balancing brain chemicals that are involved in both pain and mood regulation. For some people, these medications can make a meaningful difference by reducing pain and improving emotional well-being.

Other antidepressants, like tricyclic antidepressants (TCAs), such as amitriptyline and nortriptyline, have also been shown to help with both pain and sleep issues. However, like any medication, they come with potential side effects, such as drowsiness or weight gain, which you should be aware of before making a decision. If you're hesitant about antidepressants, it may help to have an open conversation with your healthcare provider about your concerns and explore whether this option is a good fit for you.

Anti-seizure Medications - Medications like gabapentin (Neurontin) and pregabalin (Lyrica) are often used to manage nerve-related pain, and they can be effective for some people with fibromyalgia. These medications work by calming overactive nerve signals and reducing the pain associated with central sensitization.

While they've been shown to improve pain for many, they may not be suitable for everyone. Common side effects include dizziness, fatigue, and weight gain. If you choose to explore these options, it's important to work closely with your doctor to monitor how you're feeling and adjust the dosage as needed.

Muscle Relaxants - Muscle relaxants, such as cyclobenzaprine (Flexeril), may be recommended for people who experience muscle stiffness and spasms alongside fibromyalgia. These medications can help relieve tension and discomfort in the muscles, which may improve your ability

CHAPTER 2

Medications

When it comes to managing fibromyalgia pain, there are a variety of options, and medication is one of them. However, it's important to understand that medication is not the only path, nor is it the right choice for everyone. The decision to take medication is deeply personal, and what works for one person may not work for another. That said, it's crucial to be aware of the different types of medications available, so you can make an informed choice that aligns with your own values, needs, and comfort level.

Medications can be helpful in reducing pain and improving quality of life, but they are just one piece of the puzzle. For some, they offer significant relief and make it possible to engage more fully in daily life. For others, the side effects or concerns about long-term use might outweigh the benefits. The key is finding what feels right for you—and what supports your overall health and well-being.

Pain Relievers - For many people with fibromyalgia, over-the-counter (OTC) pain relievers, such as acetaminophen (Tylenol) or nonsteroidal anti-inflammatory drugs (NSAIDs) like ibuprofen (Advil, Motrin), can provide relief from mild to moderate pain. These medications are often the first step in managing pain, and for some, they are enough to reduce discomfort and help with day-to-day functioning.

However, it's important to keep in mind that these medications are often less effective for the kind of widespread, chronic pain typical of fibromyalgia. Since fibromyalgia pain stems from how the brain processes pain, these pain relievers may not address the root cause of the discomfort. But if you find them helpful, they can be part of a broader strategy for managing pain—just be sure to use them with caution and follow your healthcare provider's advice on dosage and frequency.

radiates from their muscles or joints. It's not uncommon to feel like your whole body is bruised, or like you've been hit by a truck, even after a good night's sleep. The pain can also fluctuate—on some days it may be barely noticeable, and on others, it can be completely debilitating.

For many people with fibromyalgia, pain isn't just a physical symptom—it affects everything. It can influence your mood, your energy, and even your ability to carry out simple daily tasks. You might struggle to get out of bed in the morning, have difficulty sitting or standing for long periods of time, or find that your work and social life are impacted by the unpredictability of flare-ups. Because the pain is chronic, it can also contribute to mental exhaustion, creating a cycle where pain leads to stress, and stress leads to more pain.

The pain of fibromyalgia can also come with a sense of isolation. Since the symptoms are invisible to others, it can be hard for those around you to fully understand the extent of your discomfort. Friends and family may see you looking "fine" on the outside and might not realize that your body is crying out for relief. This can leave you feeling frustrated, misunderstood, and disconnected—compounding the emotional toll of living with chronic pain.

While the pain of fibromyalgia can feel overwhelming at times, it's important to remember that it is manageable. The first step is acknowledging that the pain is not just "in your head," but a real, physiological response. Understanding this can help you feel less defeated by it. There are several effective pain management strategies you can explore to help reduce the intensity and frequency of your pain, and through consistent practice, you can regain a sense of control over your body. In the following sections, we'll look at specific techniques—from mindfulness practices and medication options and alternative treatments—that can help you manage your pain and bring relief when you need it most.

Chapter 2

Managing My Pain

Fibromyalgia pain is unlike any other kind of pain. It's persistent, widespread, and often feels like it has no clear cause. For many people, the pain is the hardest part of living with fibromyalgia. It can affect any part of your body at any time, making it feel like a constant companion that never quite leaves. But understanding the nature of this pain is the first step toward managing it.

At its core, fibromyalgia pain is caused by an abnormal response to pain signals in the brain and nervous system. Normally, your body experiences pain as a response to an injury or irritation, and your brain processes it accordingly. But in people with fibromyalgia, the brain and spinal cord process pain signals in an amplified way. What should be mild discomfort can feel like intense, burning, or throbbing pain. This is called "central sensitization"—essentially, your nervous system becomes hyper-sensitive and reacts more strongly than it should to normal stimuli.

This pain can show up in a variety of ways. You might feel deep, aching muscles that never seem to relax, or your joints might feel stiff and tender, as if they're swollen even when they aren't. Some people experience sharp, shooting pains or a sensation of "burning" that

This book is a guide to helping you manage the most common symptoms of fibromyalgia—and to empower you with practical, actionable steps you can start taking right now to feel better. These steps aren't about curing fibromyalgia—unfortunately, there's no magic pill for that. But they are about making choices that can reduce the pain, calm the fatigue, and bring you back to yourself.

Each chapter will focus on a different area of your health and well-being that plays a key role in managing fibromyalgia. From understanding how pain impacts your body, to exploring the healing power of diet, to embracing exercise and sleep as part of your recovery, this book offers you tools to begin feeling better, day by day. The goal isn't perfection. It's progress. Small, sustainable changes that add up to a significant difference over time.

While your fibromyalgia journey is unique to you, remember that there is hope. The changes you make can lead to a life that's more manageable, more joyful, and more centered in your own power. Together, we'll explore the symptoms, challenges, and tools that can help you create your own blueprint. It's time to take the first step. Let's begin this journey to building a blueprint toward healing and empowerment.

Chapter 1

Introduction

Living with fibromyalgia can feel like carrying a weight that no one else can see. It's not just physical pain—it's the fatigue, the brain fog, the tenderness in your body that seems to never go away. The unpredictability can make you feel like you're constantly fighting a battle, but it's a battle that can feel isolated. You're not alone in this, though, and the first step toward managing fibromyalgia is understanding it—and understanding that there is hope for better days ahead.

Fibromyalgia is a chronic condition that affects the way your brain and nervous system process pain signals, amplifying them and turning what should be mild discomfort into excruciating pain. But the pain isn't the whole story. Fibromyalgia impacts many areas of life: sleep patterns, mental clarity, mood, and even the digestive system. It's a condition that varies from person to person, often making it feel like an invisible monster that only you can feel but no one else can see. You might find yourself wondering, Why does this keep happening to me? Why can't I just feel normal again? And those are valid questions. But here's the good news: it's possible to make changes that can lessen the severity of these symptoms and improve your quality of life.

Avoid Stimulants	28
Reduce Stress	29
Meditation	29
Listening to Music	30
Magnesium Sulfate Bath Soak	30
Moving Forward: Sleep as a Priority	31
Chapter 6	32
Conclusion	32
Chapter 7	34
Resources	34

Contents

Chapter 1	1
Introduction	1
Chapter 2	3
Managing My Pain	3
Medications	5
Holistic Medicines	8
Empowering Your Healing Journey	10
Other Therapies for Managing Fibromyalgia Pain	11
Not a Single Approach	14
Chapter 3	15
Diet Is Key	15
Finding Your Triggers: What Works and What Doesn't	16
Best Diets for Fibromyalgia: Reducing Inflammation	18
Nutrition and Supplements: Supporting Your Body from Within	19
A Proactive Approach	20
Chapter 4	21
Stretching and Exercise	21
Daily Stretching Your Muscles	22
The Power of Consistency	24
Chapter 5	26
Sleep	26
Environment	27
Regular Exercise	28

Copyright © 2024 by M K Higgins

All rights reserved. No part of this publication may be reproduced, stored or transmitted in any form or by any means, electronic, mechanical, photocopying, recording, scanning, or otherwise without written permission from the publisher. It is illegal to copy this book, post it to a website, or distribute it by any other means without permission.

M K Higgins asserts the moral right to be identified as the author of this work.

M K Higgins has no responsibility for the persistence or accuracy of URLs for external or third-party Internet Websites referred to in this publication and does not guarantee that any content on such Websites is, or will remain, accurate or appropriate.

Designations used by companies to distinguish their products are often claimed as trademarks. All brand names and product names used in this book and on its cover are trade names, service marks, trademarks and registered trademarks of their respective owners. The publishers and the book are not associated with any product or vendor mentioned in this book. None of the companies referenced within the book have endorsed the book.

First edition

This book was professionally typeset on Reedsy.
Find out more at reedsy.com

M K HIGGINS

Fibromyalgia: Journey to Healing

Transforming Your Pain Through Diet, Exercise, and Lifestyle Changes.